# 7 Secrets a Fit Mama Used to Lose the Baby Weight

*Things You Need to Know that "They" Don't Tell You*

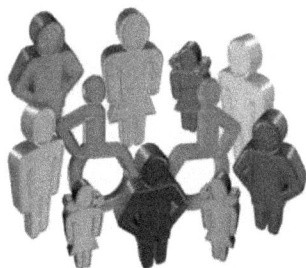

## Karla and Rich Walker

# DEDICATION

This book is dedicated to truly "good people"-our six children: Imani Vera Walker, Azaan Rich Walker, Wisdom Love Walker, Honor Courage Walker, Excellence Success Walker and Brilliant Victorious Walker

# CONTENTS

# ACKNOWLEDGMENTS

We would like to acknowledge Vera Ford, Harold Guidry, Bennie Hampton, Sharron Hampton and Jeanette Pittmon. Your unconditional love and support is tremendously appreciated. Words can only express a mere fraction of our love and gratitude for each of you.

# 1

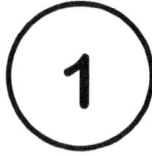

# WHAT MADE KARLA CHANGE HER BODY CAN CHANGE YOUR BODY TOO?

## BY KARLA WALKER

Defining moments have confronted you throughout your life. Some of these defining moments instantly gave you clear options; options like, stay or leave, remain silent or speak up. While other defining moments did not become apparent to you until it was too late. Regardless of where you live in the world, your race or national origin, your economic or marital status, you will have defining moments confront you and present you with options to make a decision. Your task will be to know what is best for you. Your decision will be a turning point that will challenge you to act.

It would be nice if you knew in advance that you would have glowing support of cheering friends and family once you acted on a life changing decision. But, the reality is that most life changing decisions will be greeted with raised eye brows and disparaging comments. This experience could make you doubt yourself and the relationship you have with the people you entrusted to share your decision. Nevertheless, defining moments will confront you and you will have an opportunity to change.

A defining moment confronted me after I was pregnant with my fourth son and sixth child that my husband, Rich, and I conceived together. Similarly to my pregnancies with my other boys, I was nauseous (incidentally, I experienced very little nausea during my pregnancies with my daughters, but I was really fatigued). My nausea subsided after the first trimester, and I became active again. I even began jogging, which I thought was great for me being a busy pregnant mom.

However, fatigue began to stop me in my tracks during the middle of my second trimester. Test results revealed I had pregnancy-related anemia. Before I knew it, I willfully surrendered to this energy- killing monster called anemia and stopped jogging. This was a decision I would soon regret as my

1

plans of walking instead of jogging did not happen and my plans of doing body weight exercises in the house did not happen either. And, before I knew it, my anemia seemed to worsen, and I began to struggle with debilitating low back pain, pregnancy hypertension, constipation and other discomforts.

Miraculously, my health was stable enough to give birth, naturally, in an alternative birth center. Like his five other siblings, our son's birth was without medication, peaceful and full of love as he entered the world. He latched immediately to breastfeed and was completely healthy.

However, my health after his birth was another story.

While at the hospital, I was closely monitored as my blood pressure remained unstable and headaches caused by my blood pressure would come and go. I had intense muscle cramps while in the hospital and digestive issues. With the exception of the muscle cramps, my less than optimal health after birth continued. One could say, "Karla you just gave birth to your sixth child-no worries"! But, I was worried. See, I know what it feels like to start off a pregnancy in good shape and to remain active throughout pregnancy. I know the energy and strength a healthy pregnant woman feels, even after birth. I knew in my gut the condition that being inactive for the majority of my pregnancy had put me in.

My once active lifestyle; coupled with, my vibrant and jovial spirit was now laden with concerns about my health moving forward. I thought to myself, there are so many mothers who abandon the notion of being active once they have one child. Perhaps, I needed to just accept the fact that being an overweight, inactive, mother of six children with "normal" western health problems (hypertension, constipation, etc.) was just my new lot in life. After all, I had healthy, loving kids, a good husband, a roof over our heads, nice clothes on our backs and food to eat. Maybe, I should just be thankful for all of the good things I had and have going for me and join the crowd. Though, I said nothing, *a defining moment had confronted me when I entertained these suggestions.*

Well, a little while later, my gastrointestinal issues catapulted me from uncomfortable to unbearable! As I sat in the bathroom feeling like I needed surgery for an entire digestive system transplant; I became determined *not* to spend another day like this! I immediately began taking action. I was exclusively breastfeeding our two month old infant son at the time; so, I was mindful that any method I used had to be both safe for my son and effective for me to get positive results. To make a long story short, I started a new and strategic eating regimen and exercise routine. Wow! My gastrointestinal issues seemed to be resolving themselves as I continued to exercise along with my new eating regimen. I was hooked!

I felt a jaw-dropping improvement within a few short weeks. After a while, I was healed-thankfully. So, I asked myself, "should I stop eating this way and decrease my exercise? After all, I am feeling better. A "no" answer resounded in the depths of my soul. No, I should not stop eating this way nor should I decrease my physical activity. In fact, I should get more active and set bigger health and fitness goals. And, this is exactly what I started to do.

Far too often do women, especially mothers, take care of themselves *for a moment* and then immediately begin caring for everyone else. However, ladies, we need to love ourselves without guilt and recognize the defining moments that confront us.

# 2

## STICKS AND STONES

### BY RICH & KARLA WALKER

*I CAN.*

*Did is a word of achievement, Won't is a word of retreat, Might is a word of bereavement, Can't is a word of defeat, Ought is a word of duty, Try is a word each hour, Will is a word of beauty, Can is a word of power. –Author Unknown*

The words you say about yourself will cause you to be empowered or disempowered, succeed or fail, overcome or be overwhelmed. Your words will affect you in every area of your life and health and fitness is no different. Every aspect of you is a culmination of what you have said about yourself. The words that others have spoken to you may have helped to form the words you believe about yourself, but it is the words you to believe about yourself that makes the difference in your life.

How do you know what you believe? Just listen to the words you say about yourself. What do you say about yourself if you make a mistake? Do you say things like, "I'm so stupid!" "I can't do anything right!" How about when you do not get the results that you were expecting. Do you say things like, "I can't make good decisions?" I just don't know how to make anything work!" What do you say about yourself when you misspeak or your words to others come out the wrong way? Do you say things like, "I'm such an idiot -don't listen to me!" "Please forgive me; I don't know what I am talking about!" And, if after a break-up of a marriage, friendship or romantic relationship, do you say things, such as, "I'm not worth keeping, I guess."

If you are not careful, this self-defeated talk can transfer to your children or your partner. The words you say about yourself as a person, a mom, etc. are important. You may think that you are just saying words and that it is no big deal. After all, sticks and stones can break your bones, but *words* can never

4

hurt you-right? Wrong! Words either lay a foundation for *success*, failure, defeat or victory.

The words you say about regaining your figure after childbirth is like an umbilical cord; and, the words you believe about regaining your figure after childbirth is like the placenta to your baby. Meaning, your words are critical to the overall life and vitality of your fitness program. This sounds so serious because it is vital. Many people who do not reach or maintain their fitness goals erroneously think the reason was due to *the time* their family member or friend offered them their favorite indulgence; or *the time* they went on vacation; or the "such and such" party that had all of that good food. But, it is likely that a person not reaching or no longer maintaining their fitness goals started at the time they believed and spoke self-defeated talk about themselves and fitness program.

Now, with all this said, one of the most common self-defeating conversation pieces moms have with themselves and other moms is that about their body. A mom may say, "Girl, you know I put my 'fat butt' in my van and cleared out the clearance section!" Or, "Girl, who needs a jacket when you have 'thunder thighs' like mine-I'm 'bout to start a fire over here". Whether talking about having a turkey neck or blowing in the wind arms or everything in between, self-defeating talk affects you, your effort to achieve results in your fitness program, and your family, especially your kids who do as you do.

Unfortunately, mothers often really hit below the belt when they compare their bodies with other mothers' bodies. Oh, I wish I had a "thigh gap" like super model..., I wish I had a booty like singer..., and the disparaging comments go on and on.

But, be encouraged, understanding that your body type and body shape is beautiful in its own right. Set yourself free from the pressure to be a good copy of someone else, and learn to be an excellent original of you. Embrace the type of body you were born with-then smile.

So, your words will either put you in a mind-set to succeed or fail. This is great news because your words are something you can change. In contrast, if the success of your fitness program depended on something like, the color of your skin, gender, age or your ethnicity, then you would be in big trouble;

however, the success of your fitness program begins with what you SAY about the success of your fitness program. Starting right now, you can change what you say about you, your body and the fitness results you will get moving forward.

Finally, stay encouraged! Let's see what our little birdie R.O.B.I.N has to share.

~Remember Your Time to have a Rocking Optimal Body is Now! ~

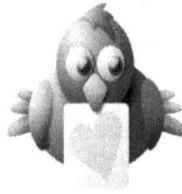

**Karla and Rich's Personal Training Tip #1:** Fit Mamas speak motivating words about their fitness efforts.

**BOOK BONUS: Mom-Minded Fitness Plan #1**: In order to help bring life and not death to your fitness efforts- Get a ream of tape that you can write on, like beige masking tape. Write one motivating word about your fitness program on a piece of tape. Place that piece of tape, with your one motivating fitness word on it, to something that you look at throughout the day, such as your mobile phone or tablet. Feel free to ask your children for one encouraging word you can write on the tape-provided that your children are old enough to talk.

This easy to do tip can safe guard you against the type of discouragement that makes you want to quit and be a yo-yo dieter. It also sets the stage for your children to be healthy and have a positive self-image.

# 3

## THE POWER OF KNOWING

### BY RICH WALKER

**How Does Knowing Your Body-Type and Body- Shape Empower You to Stay Motivated to Reach Your Fitness Goals and Achieve Success Easier?**

Picture this in your mind, a man named Brian working out at Sensations Health Club. Brian is a 6'2, 230lb, 8% body-fat carrying muscular man. Brian is at Sensations practically every day. He loves to improve and build his body, especially by lifting weights. And, Brian always gains muscle relatively easier than a lot of other people in Sensations Health Club. Usually, when Brian is lifting weights he feels eyes staring at him, particularly, from a man named Sam. Sam is a 6'3, 165lb slender man. Sam has had a desire to build muscle for years, but no matter how hard he tries his progress is slow as a turtle.

However, Sam has noticed that in the last three months Brian's muscles have swelled up big just like balloons do when a person puts water in them to the maximum. Sam is envious of Brian's ability to build his muscle so fast. This is why Sam is always staring at Brian when he is lifting weights. Sam watches what Brian does while lifting weights and he imitates the same weight-lifting routines that Brian performs. But, no matter how hard Sam tries, Brian's weight-lifting routines don't work for Sam the same way they work for Brian. As a result, Sam has become discouraged about exercising anymore. Sam spoke to himself and said, "What's the point? My workout program feels like I'm outside in my yard raking leaves on a windy day. No matter how hard I try, I don't get any results. Oh, but wait, I do get results. I lose weight without even trying".

Next, imagine a woman named Katie working out at Sensations Health Club. Katie is 5'6 and 220lbs. Her desire is to lose 100lbs and fit into a size four dress. Recently, Katie became secretly angry at her friend and workout partner Simone, who is 5'5 and 140lbs; because, Simone lost ten pounds and she didn't lose any weight. Also, they both go to Sensations Health Club at least five days a week together. And, they do the same exercise routine, but Katie didn't lose any weight. When Katie found out about Simone losing ten pounds she privately kicked over her kitchen table and screamed as loud as she could. Then Katie thought in her mind, "it seems that if I just look at food I gain weight. Why does Simone get all the results?"

Actually, there is a logical reason for the discrepancy of muscle gain between Brian and Sam and the weight loss between Katie and Simone. The reason is because each of the persons named have different body-types. However, not just the individuals named have different body-types, but all humans are born with one of three different body-types. The three body-types are: 1. Ectomorph. 2. Endomorph. 3. Mesomorph. Each of these three body-types has distinct characteristics. First, the ectomorph body-type is on the slimmer side. And, they were born with relatively fewer muscle cells. In addition, those with ectomorph body-types, generally, do not gain weight easily. Yet, they do lose weight relatively quickly.

Second, those with an endomorph body-type were born with relatively more fat cells. Therefore, those with an endomorph body-type naturally carry more body-fat than people who have the other two body-types. Also, those with an endomorph body-type do not lose weight easily.

Third, those with a mesomorph body-type were born with a higher number of muscle cells than those born with an ectomorph or endomorph body-type. Mesomorph body-types usually gain muscle quickly when they workout. To add, even when those with a mesomorph body-type gain weight they still have a muscular look to them. And, they burn fat relatively quick because of their larger number of muscle cells.

Next, humans were also born with one of three body shapes. The three body-shapes are: 1. The apple shape. This body shape carries more weight in the upper body. 2. The pear shape. The pear shape carries more weight in the lower body. 3. The banana shape. The banana shape equally distributes weight between the upper and lower body.

# How Can Knowing Your Body-Type And Body Shape Help You?

Well, in the case of Katie, the lady from the story earlier, she has an endomorph body-type. She was born with more fat cells. And, her friend/workout partner, Simone, has an ectomorph body-type. This body-type loses weight faster than an endomorph body-type. If Katie was aware of her and Simone's body-type then she would realize the uselessness of comparing herself with Simone. Katie would instantly know that it is an unfair comparison, in regards to the speed of weight loss, between her and Simone.

Likewise, because of Katie and Simone's unique body-types, they require different workout programs. In other words, they should not be following the same exercise program. This is because their bodies have different needs. With these things in mind, Katie would understand she has no justifiable reason to hold secret anger toward Simone because Simone lost ten pounds and she didn't. Furthermore, if Katie had knowledge of her body-type she would have a greater peace of mind when working out in the gym. This is because she would know that she is racing against herself and not the other people in the gym.

In addition, back to my other story from earlier, if Sam knew that he had an ectomorph body-type, then he probably wouldn't be envious of Brain who has a mesomorph body-type. Sam would understand that genetically people with mesomorph body-types build muscle faster than people with ectomorph body-types. Thus, the reason why Brain builds muscle faster than Sam is based on their different body-types.

Furthermore, concerning the subject of body shape, visualize a woman named Yolanda. Yolanda loves being the center of attention and having men desire her. So, she tiresomely tries to develop an hour-glass figure. Yolanda has this thought that if she eats lots of potatoes and drinks lots of milk, then she will eventually gain an hour-glass figure. But, by following the potato and milk program, Yolanda hasn't gotten the results she expects; however, Yolanda has gained weight in her arms, shoulders, back, face, and her belly. Yet, Yolanda's friend, Lorraine, eats the same way as Yolanda and she gains weight in her hips and buttock area.

The differences between where Yolanda and Lorraine gain weight is because they were born with different body-shapes. For example, Yolanda is an apple shape, and Lorraine is a pear shape. If Yolanda was aware that she had an apple body-shape, then she would know that it is aimless for her to be on a potato and milk diet for the purpose of getting an hour-glass figure. Also, if Yolanda knew she had an apple body-shape then she would realize that she is not genetically inclined to having an hour glass figure, but instead she could focus on making her apple-shaped body the best it can be.

Additionally, envision a man named Joseph. Joseph likes lifting weights, and he wants to be a professional body-builder. Currently, Joseph is pleased that his upper-body is getting bigger and more muscular, but he is gravely disappointed that his legs are small and on the skinny side. However, if Joseph was conscious that he has an apple body-shape he could be encouraged to know that it is not his effort in the gym that is causing his legs to lag behind his upper-body development, but it is because of his apple body-shape.

In contrast, Joseph's friend, Pete, has a gigantic and muscular upper body and lower body. This is because Pete has a banana shaped body. In other words, Pete's body weight is evenly distributed. With this said, if Joseph knows he has an apple body-shape and his friend Pete has a banana body-shape, he doesn't have to be discouraged that he is not getting the same results as Pete. Because he would know, that he gains weight more in his upper-body than his lower-body because he has a apple body-shape, while his friend Pete, has his weight evenly distributed across his upper-body and lower-body because he has a banana body-shape.

Accordingly, you can benefit from the examples of Brian, Sam, Katie, Simone, Yolanda, Lorraine, Joseph and Pete, when thinking about body-types and body-shapes. Specifically, there are a number of benefits that you will receive from knowing your body-type and body-shape and applying what you know in a skillful way:

1. You will enhance your exercise and nutrition program. This is because when you understand the nature of your body-type and body shape you will not have unrealistic expectations for yourself. Unrealistic expectations lead to

disappointment, and disappointment can lead to giving-up on your fitness goals.

2. You will be empowered to determine what will be an effective exercise program for you. Too many times an individual with an ectomorph body-type is trying to work-out like a person with a mesomorph body-type; similarly, to what Sam was doing with Brian, and the person with the ectomorph body-type expects the same results.

Unfortunately, in the end, this leads to discouragement. Discouragement takes the place of motivation and the fitness enthusiast is vulnerable to quitting.

3. You will be able to build an eating regimen that is compatible with you and the goals you want to reach. Hence, you can avoid the common disappointment that happens when people do not get the results they are looking for because they are following exercise and eating programs that are not conducive for their body-type and body shape.

4. You can formulate fitness goals that are realistic and achievable for you, instead of coming up with goals that are compatible with people that have different body-types and body shapes than yourself.

Remember, it is always best to set goals that are achievable. Also, you want to be able to see progress as you move along your fitness program. But, if you set unachievable goals for yourself your progress will be stagnant. With this said…

~Remember Your Time to have a Rocking Optimal Body is Now! ~

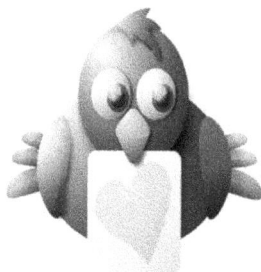

**Karla and Rich's Personal Training Tip #2:** Fit Mamas that learn their body-type and body-shape are better equipped to get results.

**Book Bonus: Mom-Minded Fitness Plan ##2:** In order to avoid discouragement, make fitness and nutritional motivational tools for yourself. For example, get a large poster board. Put a current picture of yourself and children on the left side of the poster board with the date underneath the current picture. Also, put your current measurements of your waist, hips, thighs, arms, etc. under the picture. On the right side of the poster board put a line with the date -30 days from the date of the poster. On top of the right side, put your name-with the words: "You Can Do It" beneath your name. And, have your kids and partner write encouraging phrases to you. Lastly, on the right side of the poster, put the measurements that you are seeking to attain in thirty days. Put this poster board in a place you will see it daily. Also, you can continue to use this strategy for 60 days, 90 days, etc. Again, this is one example of a motivational tool that you can use.

# 4

## WEARING WHITE OUT OF SEASON

### BY RICH WALKER

The results you receive from working-out and dieting will produce a unique look because of your given body-type and body-shape that will likely be different than other people's body-types and body shapes. Thus, no matter how hard you exercise your look will fit into the parameters of your own body-type and body shape. Therefore, it is effective to focus your attention on making your body-type and body shape the best that it can be.

As a result of this mindset, following your fitness program will be much more desirable and easier compared to operating outside your genetic boundaries.

Frankly, one of the biggest obstacles that people encounter when trying to accomplish a fitness goal is following an exercise and nutrition program that is outside their genetic boundaries. The thing that makes this obstacle so problematic is that it is invisible to the naked eye. In other words, people do not know that this problem exists. The person may know that there is a problem because they are not achieving the goals they desire, but they are looking in the wrong places.

For instance, the person that is not getting positive results in their fitness program may blame their personal trainer's advice or criticize the diet plan they are following as faulty, to name a few. But, in reality, the problem is that the given person is trying to achieve a fitness goal outside of their genetic boundaries. The person is neglecting to apply sound principles in relation to their body-type and body-shape.

How do you determine what your body-type and body shape is? You can determine what your body-type is by traveling to the past in your mind. Specifically, focus on your life from 10 years old and below. Begin to analyze what your body was like during that time-frame. Were you on the slim side? Did you eat a lot, but did not gain weight easily? If the answer is yes to these questions you likely have an ectomorph body-type. Or were you chubby and gained weight easily? If this is the case, then you have an endomorph body-type. Or did you naturally have a muscular frame? If your answer is yes to this question, you likely have a mesomorph body-type.

Also, just because you are overweight or obese does not automatically mean you have an endomorph body-type. As an example, it is possible for any of the three body-types to become overweight or obese. But, each of the body-types has a different look. For instance, the person with a mesomorph body-type will look muscular and solid when they are overweight or obese. The person with an endomorph body-type looks natural and in their real state when overweight or obese. In contrast, the person with an ectomorph body-type looks less natural when they are overweight or obese, as though they are not in their real state.

Now, let's talk about the body-shapes. How do you know your body-shape? First, if you carry most of your weight in your upper-body; then, you have an apple body-shape. Second, if you carry most of your weight in your lower-body; then, you have a pear body-shape. Third, if you carry your weight equally in your upper-body and lower-body; then, you have a banana body-shape.

In conclusion, knowing your body-type and body shape will empower you to keep motivated to achieve success easier in your workout routine. However, just the opposite will likely be true if you construct your fitness program without knowledge of your body-type and body shape and your chances of failure increase. Karla has a good analogy between the fashion world and the fitness world: "To some, it is unfashionable to wear white colored clothing during the fall and winter seasons. It is not an option to be out of season in the fashion world. Likewise, in the fitness world, it should not be an option to set fitness goals outside the parameters or ability of your genetic make-up". So, what is secret number three?

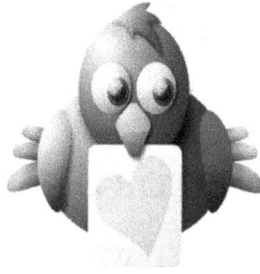

**Karla and Rich's Personal Training Tip #3:** Fit Mamas set goals for their body-type and body-shape.

**Book Bonus: Mom-Minded Fitness Plan #3:** In order to achieve a goal that is attainable for your given body-type and shape, try this: Identify the most outstanding asset of your body. You will be accentuating the positive! Focus on the most beautiful asset of your body by committing to doing three exercises, thirty repetitions each, three days a week, for thirty days. Regarding your least favorite asset, commit to doing two exercises, twenty repetitions, two days a week, for twenty days. This routine can help reinforce you to focus more on highlighting the beauty of your specific body-type and body-shape, while still exercising and embracing the beauty of your entire body.

# MIRROR-MIRROR ON THE WALL

## BY RICH WALKER

### Why Do Some People that Workout *Always* Win the Prize of Accomplishing Their Fitness Dreams While Others Fall Short?

Do you have fitness goals that you want to accomplish, but you always fall short of achievement? And, why do some people always reach their fitness dreams? Socrates, the Greek Philosopher, can help lead us to the answer.

Socrates said, "An unexamined life is not worth living". This is an insightful statement that applies to everyday life. Yet, not only does it apply to everyday life, but it also applies to your exercise and diet plan. To put it differently, an unexamined exercise and nutrition program is not worth following! Why is this statement true?

The general protocol of a medical doctor in relation to his or her patient can illuminate us on why an unexamined exercise and diet plan is not worth following. For instance, prior to Dr. Jennifer Wallace giving her patient, Amanda, a *diagnosis* and *prescription* to treat her high blood pressure, Dr. Wallace did a thorough examination to determine the cause of Amanda's discomfort.

Just the opposite, Dr. Wallace would have demonstrated incompetency, if she would have given Amanda a treatment without, first, giving her a careful examination. Why? The answer is because without a proper exam Dr. Wallace's conclusion would be considered a guess, and guesses are *not* always reliable.

Likewise, when you don't carefully examine your exercise and diet plan it is unreliable! The physical bodies of humans are similar in many respects, but, at the same time, human's bodies are also unique. Therefore, Plan A (a given exercise and nutrition program) may work in some ways for you, but in other ways Plan A is useless for you. This is an example of why it is so important to exam your exercise and diet plan while you are following it. If examination is not done, there is a higher potential for disappointment to start knocking at your door because you have falling short of reaching your fitness dreams. However, when you regularly examine your exercise and diet program, you will make faster improvements in your body and your overall health.

With all this said, what exactly does examining your exercise and diet plan mean? It means that daily, you pay close attention to how your body is responding to your exercise and diet program. What does this daily routine look like? It is revealed in the following list:

1.  Document what you eat and what times you eat.

2.  Document how you feel after eating the food you consume.

3.  Document how you feel after the exercises you perform.

4.  Document how your body is responding to your exercise and diet plan in terms of how it looks and your overall physical performance.

5.  Take time to think carefully about what may not be working in your exercise and diet plan.

6.  Evaluate how you can improve upon your exercise and diet program.

7.  Immediately take action on your discoveries found in number five and six of this list.

In contrast, based on all this information, can you see how an unexamined exercise and diet plan is not worth following? Surely, time will be wasted and disappointment will be experienced, if you follow an exercise and diet plan without regular examination of it. Of course, this is because you could be continuously repeating the wrong actions that could lead to limited or no positive fitness results.

~Remember Your Time to have a Rocking Optimal Body is Now! So, what is secret number four?

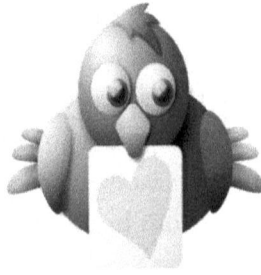

**Karla and Rich's Personal Trainers Tip #4:** Fit Mamas gladly examine their fitness routine and make adjustments as needed to keep their fitness program productive and result oriented.

**Book Bonus: Karla's Action Plan #4:** Get a new notebook and a kids art set if your kids are two years old or older. Make this notebook into a fitness journal for you to examine your fitness routines and nutritional intake. Invite your children to decorate your fitness journal. This can help rally their support and investment in your fitness and nutritional program. If your children are not old enough to contribute at this, feel free to share your decorated journal with your partner, family or close friend to help rally their support and investment.

# (6)

## WHAT'S ON YOUR AGENDA

### BY KARLA WALKER

Mothers of all ages and national origins tend to put everyone else on their agenda but themselves. Truth: some mothers only put themselves on their agenda for special occasions, like their birthday or an infrequent girl's night out. However, doing something for them on a regular basis just doesn't happen. This type of mother often has healthy and happy children and partner; yet, her health and even sometime her happiness may suffer.

You are just as important as the task your boss is asking you to complete. You are just as important as your kids needing you to do "x, y, and z". You are just as important as the errand your spouse or significant other wants you to do a.s.a.p. You are just as important as the phone call you need to make or place you need to take your friend and family member. You, your wants and needs are important.

So...often, we as moms try to be all things to all people only to fail at being anything to ourselves. We try to please our spouse/partner, our kids, our boss, our family, our friends, our children's teacher, and more. Soon it is time for you to go to bed, wake up, and do it all over again. Inevitably, you may begin to feel that you are pulled in so many directions that you are not being your best for all those you are trying to please, and you certainly are not being your best for yourself.

In this moment that you begin to feel this way, take a pause. Examine yourself. Examine your health and fitness program. Scan your priorities. Honestly, identify where you fall on your list of priorities. If you are high on this list of priorities, then keep doing what you are doing. However, you may have fallen into the "mom-hole", if your needs, wants, desires are low or the lowest on your priority list. What is a 'mom-hole', you may ask? A mom-hole is like a man-hole. As you know, a manhole is an underground chamber used for many different reasons, such as having an access point for making

19

connections, inspection, valve adjustments or performing maintenance on underground public utilities. This includes sewers, telephone, electricity, storm drains, and heating/gas for city districts. Needless to say, it is a lot happening under the surface.

In like manner, there is a lot happening in our lives as moms. There can be an internal busyness within a mom to feel as though she must juggle everything. This internal busyness can feel like she is in a deep hole-hence, a "mom-hole". So, whether you look at the mom who dropped off another delicious pound cake for the Parent/Teacher social; or the mom who scowls as she is late picking up her child from school-there is often a lot happening underneath the surface of a loving moms smile or scowl. Either of the two types of moms can be in a 'mom-hole'.

Well, manholes and mom-holes have to be inspected or EXAMINED frequently, otherwise the steam and pressure can build from all of the activity happening beneath the surface and the top could blow causing someone to get hurt. The fact that you are investing in reading this book tells us that you value being a happy and healthy mom who is good to others and herself. Thus, stay encouraged as you take examination of your overall priorities very seriously.

If you find that you need to move yourself up higher on your priority list-then do it. Confidently, embrace the fact that you are just as important as many of the items on your "to-do" list. This includes your health and fitness.

Fortunately, taking time to examine and improve your health and fitness through exercise will:

1. Increase your energy levels and serotonin in your brain, which can lead to improvement in your focus on all that you must do.

2. Release endorphins into your bloodstream causing you to feel much more energized throughout the day.

3. Make family time more fun. You will have more stamina to spend time with your kids at the park, swimming, playing hide-and-seek or tag.

4. Give you a bridge to better relationships. You can exercise with a spouse or a friend.

5. Slow or help prevent heart disease, stroke, high blood pressure, high cholesterol, type 2 diabetes, arthritis, osteoporosis (bone loss), and loss of muscle mass.

6. Strengthen your heart, thus making your life feel easier to manage.

7. Allows you to eat more of your favorite treats, in moderation of course. Muscle burns more calories at rest than body fat. So, the more muscle you have the higher your resting metabolic rate will be. And, you will also burn more calories while you're actually exercising.

8. Improve your mama flare! Over time, exercise consistently will strengthen your muscles, increase flexibility, and improve your overall performance and flare to be mom. And, finally...

9. Shed that unwanted pooch from child birth more quickly.

Lastly, understand that your health and fitness is a part of you. Your hair and nails looking pretty and your make-up being flawless all losses its importance if you are looking good in a hospital bed. Again, your health and fitness is a part of you. So, examine your life and your health and fitness program. Make adjustments where necessary.

~Remember Your Time to have a Rocking Optimal Body is Now! ~

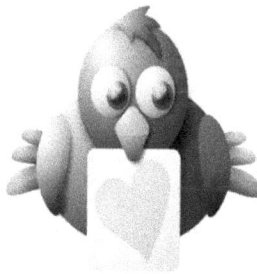

**Karla and Rich's Personal Training Tip #5:** Fit Mamas make it a priority to put themselves on their agenda.

**Book Bonus: Mom-Minded Fitness Plan #5:** Ask your child or children to use their skills to make a "happy place" for you. If they are young, you may want to suggest for them to make a princess castle or tent in the house (made using various blankets). If you have an infant, then ask your partner to use their skills to make a "happy place" for you, such as setting up a certain area in the house a particular way. And, if you really want your happy place to be special, then let your partner know that you will make a romantic happy place for the both of you after they do this for you.

**This next part is IMPORTANT!** Ask your children or your partner what time and duration each day you can go to the 'happy place' they made for you? Again, you will need their support and investment so that your time to make yourself a priority is respected. Lastly, DO NOT let this time to be changed once it is set, unless a life or death emergency occurs. Why? As mothers we tend to be so accommodating that we accommodate ourselves right out of our agenda for the day. This can no longer happen if you truly want to be a fit mama. One of the essential ways a Fit mama's body transforms is by them making themselves- their run – their yoga practice- etc. a fixed priority. You doing this action plan will send an excellent message that it is o.k. to love and respect yourself while you love and respect others.

Finally, once a happy place is created and a time is set, use it to stretch, meditate, examine your progress, or just to be happy. Smile. You are on the right path-Fit Mama!

# (7)

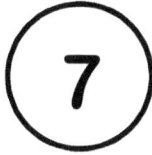

## WISH UPON A STAR

BY KARLA WALKER

As moms, we are well familiar with Walt Disney and the famous song written by **Songwriters Ned Washington and Leigh Hairline** that says,

"When you wish upon a star

Makes no difference who you are

Anything your heart desires

Will come to you

If your heart is in your dream

No request is too extreme

When you wish upon a star

As dreamers do

Fate is kind

She brings to those to love

The sweet fulfillment of

Their secret longing

Like a bolt out of the blue

Fate steps in and sees you through

When you wish upon a star

Your dreams come true

In many ways, humans are generally dreamers. We dream of a better job, a better car, a better house, etc. As mothers we often want to carry on these dreams for our kids, so *they* can have a better childhood and life than our own. We tend to defer to our children and not ourselves as though there is something terrible about wanting dreams for ourselves after becoming a mom. Where does this thinking come from? I will share where it comes from for me.

I grew up with two loving parents who worked while raising my brother and me. Both are retired now, but my dad was a hardworking factory worker and my mom was a medical biller for a local hospital. Both of my parents have a mindset that parents should do anything for their kids; that is safe and legal of course. Ha! Seriously though, they believe that parents should sacrifice and even go without so their kids will have what they need and want. I believe my mom privately feels as though this selfless philosophy applies more to her than my dad because she is the mom and that is what good moms do.

There are many moms who identify with my mom. Like me, the children of such a mother are not without typical childhood or adolescent issues, but through any issues, the children most often know that- they know- they are truly loved. I know I felt loved as a child and I still do feel this love as an adult by my parents.

Yet, the challenge of this philosophy is that *without balance*, the healthy concept of thoughtful parenting becomes blurred with the unhealthy concept of self-slaughter parenting. What is self-slaughter parenting? Simply explained, it is a parenting style where the parent does so much for their kids that they stay stressed-out over their children, which causes health problems and an early grave. For example, slaughtering animals does not acknowledge the animal. The animal's rights and feelings are not considered. Likewise, some mothers, parent in such a way that their rights and feelings are not acknowledged and considered, even something as simple as the mother's right to privacy to use the bathroom by themselves may be violated. For instance, I personally enjoy privacy in the bathroom. I am not a woman who must ask their friend to join them to a trip to the commode. That may be for some, just not for me. Yet, I use to think it was absolutely necessary for our children to go in the bathroom with me if they wanted.

One day I left the house to take care of something, and I left my husband and children at home. My husband uses the bathroom without the children. So, I asked if the children went to the bathroom with him while I was gone. He looked at me as though I said his favorite basketball player was the worst player in the NBA. It was something about my husband's resounding "no" that made it click to me. The children were ok and he was ok if our children did not violate my husband's privacy. I felt surprised and free! Free to love my children and free to have my own preferences, such as using the bathroom alone if I like.

One may say, "What is the problem with putting your children's needs before your own? Nothing is wrong with it as long as you do not do this all of the time. Yes, we need more people in this world who think deeply about others, especially children. But, we also need more people who think deeply about themselves. I am not talking about thinking more deeply about ones' self in the way that is superficial, egotistical, and borderline narcissistic. That way hurts people. Instead, I am meaning to think more deeply about yourself so you can cater to your needs the way you cater to the needs of your children.

You are mindful of their needs, you listen to their needs/ preferences, and you make adjustments because you love them. In the same manner, be mindful of your physical needs. Listen to the needs and preferences of your body and make adjustments, such as changing your diet or your level of physical activity. And, do this because you love yourself.

You showing this type of love towards yourself can lead you to better health and faster weight loss results. Now, that is good news.

As mothers, we should show a love toward ourselves that is kind, patient, forgiving, understanding and empowering. Showing this kind of love towards ourselves will help us to better love our children, partner and others. Showing this kind of love towards ourselves is necessary to have a successful fitness program.

How? Well, the love it takes to make sacrifices for your children, even when you are tired or busy, is the same love you will need to make sacrifices for yourself when you are tired or busy. This is the kind of love that good dreams are full of! Dreams give us hope. Dreams are limitless. Like the song says: 'if your heart is in your dream-no request is too extreme'.

You have to tap into the dreamer within you in order to be a Fit Mama. Fit mama's have the audacity to dare to dream for a better body and better health. And, Fit Mamas love themselves with a balanced nurturing love that allows them to dream for *better* in the first place. So, in the midst of seeing flabby mid-sections on most all non-celebrity moms, and being told by society, grandmothers, moms, sisters, aunts, etc., that your body goes downhill after having kids; a Fit mama dreams of a better body. A fit mama has the audacity to believe and actual say:

> "I can have a better body!
>
> I can be in better health.
>
> My booty can look better in my jeans.
>
> I can be, and I can have better dog-gone-it!"

Yes, it will take a lot of nerve on your part to dream for different results with your body after having children. But, the healthy love you have for yourself will give you the nerve you need. Truth be told, you have some love for yourself right now to be reading this book.

Lastly, the song says, "Like a bolt out of the blue-Fate steps in and sees you through." The love you have for yourself will see you through to your dream body and fitness goals. It will help you look forward to tomorrow, as it is another chance to improve on your eating regimen and fitness goals. And, it will help you truly believe in greater possibilities for your physical body to achieve. Do not let your age, number of kids you have, how many responsibilities you have, stop you from improving yourself and accomplishing your fitness goals.

# 8

## NOTORIOUS C

BY RICH WALKER

**Uncover How You Can *Triumph* Over This Notorious Enemy That Has Your Exercise And Diet Program In A Head-Lock**

There is a notorious enemy that wants to keep you stuck in the mud concerning your exercise and diet program. This enemy wants to prevent you from experiencing the joy that would come by you looking in the mirror and seeing the body image of your dreams. It is as if this enemy has your exercise and diet program in a head-lock, and your exercise and diet program cannot break free. Who is this enemy?

The notorious enemy being described is revealed in the following example: Imagine two men named Joey and Andy. Joey is 5'10 and 320lbs and Andy is 6'0 and 340lbs. Both of these men have loved to eat all their life. In fact, tomorrow is the local "Who Can Eat the Most Ribs Contest" at Porky's Pig Hut. The winner wins a three-month supply of ribs, pig feet, pork bacon, and ham hocks. So, Andy asked Joey, "Hey, man, are you ready for the rib contest tomorrow. I know I'm going to beat you and everybody else. I've been practicing." Joey replied, "I'm not going to the rib contest tomorrow. I'm on a new diet and exercise program." Andy laughed so hard at Joey, that while laughing, he accidently vomited his lunch all over the floor.

While Andy cleaned up the mess, he said to Joey, "Man, you were born fat, and you'll be fat the rest of your life. You've never lost weight and you have only gained weight. Why not enjoy yourself and eat what you want? Dieting and exercising is a waste of time for people like me and you. Man, come back to reality and stop being in a fantasy world. Wait until I tell the guys about this one." Joey did not like being a laughingstock, and what Andy was saying made a lot of sense to Joey. So, Joey told Andy, "Hey, maybe you're right. I probably am just fooling myself. I'm better off being and acting like the person I was born to be, and it is obvious that I was born to be a fat man that loves to eat. So, hear me loud and clear, I'll be at that rib contest tomorrow. And you won't stand a chance against me, Andy!" You have just witnessed Joey being defeated by the notorious enemy. Do you know who this enemy is, yet?

The notorious enemy is complacency. What is complacency? Complacency is having a self-satisfaction coupled with being unaware and uninformed of the deficiencies and dangers of your decision. In other words, complacency is being stuck in a rut. Also, complacency does not always play fair. It will present itself in a non-threatening and logical fashion, just how Andy presented his reasoning to Joey. For instance, complacency will attack you through the people and the things you associate with on a regular basis. Clearly, we can see that Joey was committed to his workout and diet program. But, Andy came along and discouraged him. The peer-pressure got to Joey.

The story of Joey and Andy shows that who you associate with regularly will affect your aspirations in life and this includes your exercise and diet plan. In addition, the TV shows you watch, what you read, and the organizations you belong to will also affect you. All these things named are avenues that complacency hides behind to keep you stuck in a rut. When you are stuck in a rut you are satisfied where you are (even if you are not pleased with your position) and you do not pursue anything greater. However, you can beat complacency. How?

**Here Are Several Things You Can Do To Triumph Over Complacency:**

- Communicate regularly with people that are not within your inner-circle.

- Communicate with people who have different perspectives than your own on health and nutrition.

- Communicate with people who pursue big goals concerning health and fitness.

- Read magazines and books that can expand your thinking about what you can accomplish in your health and fitness.

- Go places where you can observe and be in the atmosphere of healthy and fit people that are implementing healthy habits.

- Hang out with people that will support your health and fitness goals.

If you act on the things you have read, you can break-free from the head-lock that complacency has your exercise and diet plan in and you can body-slam complacency to its defeat in your life.

~Remember Your Time to have a Rocking Optimal Body is Now! ~

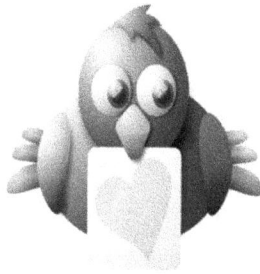

**Karla and Rich's Personal Training Tips #6:** Fit Mamas are always challenging themselves.

**Book Bonus: Mom-Minded Fitness Plan #6:** Remember that complacency is kryptonite to your body transformation dreams, so try the following: Have your children or your partner challenge you to complete a particular exercise they know or learned. You determine the "reps", which is the number of times you do the exercise continuously and the "sets", which is how many intervals you do the exercise continuously (i.e., the 'reps').

For one week, every other day, have your support system (i.e., your child, children, spouse, partner, etc.) watch you complete the exercise they challenged you to. Record how you performed. Have them put your fitness performance record in a special place, like their treasure chest. Review your results *with* your support system. Celebrate your ability to perform the exercise and brainstorm of ways to improve your performance *with* your support system. Hopefully, you will perform better each time you do the exercise challenge. If you do not improve, you can ask your support system to help you find a health and fitness professional, like a Personal Trainer. Regardless of your performance, this activity can strengthen the relationship with your support system; inspire your support system to be healthier; and it can encourage your children and partner to dream big, accept difficulties with a positive mind-set and strength to overcome.

# 9

# A FIT MAMA'S RESPECT FOR *THIS* IS THE DIFFERENCE BETWEEN THEM AND OTHER MAMAS

## BY KARLA WALKER

There will certainly be obstacles on your journey to become a fit mama, as well as staying a fit mama. It can be very disheartening to make improvements in your body, only to lose your results. No worries! Do not be overwhelmed with the fear of failure. This chapter will address and help you not fall off of the Fit Mamas Rock wagon, so to speak. Let's get into it, shall we?

RESPECT- this seven-letter word is a *must have* component in your fit program if you are going to become fit or maintain your fitness results. As you may know, respect is either a deal-maker or a deal-breaker. Whether you are talking about relationships, business, or fitness; respect goes a long way. As it relates to fitness and becoming a Fit Mama that Rocks, it is important to respect the process and the results you obtain *throughout* the process.

We as women and mothers, in general, tend to be our own worse critics in an unhealthy and disparaging way. In fact, there are some women and mothers who reinforce their familiarity with disparaging criticism by watching gossip-based television shows that are hurtful in their criticism. This familiarity with showing contempt for others and oneself will transfer to the process of becoming a fit mama. Let's look at a mother who we will call Brenda, in order to illustrate this point.

Brenda is a loving mother of 3 beautiful children. She has two action-figure imitating boys who want to be just like their dad who proudly serves in the United States Marines as a sergeant. Brenda has a tough as nails and cute as a button little daughter who holds her own as she keeps up with her older brothers. As her three children are getting older and more involved in sports, school and their friends, Brenda feels that she has more free time on her hands to exercise. Her husband stays healthy and fit all year round and is more than willing to help her when he is not serving overseas.

Brenda started exercising by walking around her neighborhood and eating more salad than pizza during Friday night movies with the kids. And, to her own surprise, Brenda stopped drinking soda pop and began drinking water like a fish. Brenda's husband and kids were very proud of her. Before long, Brenda was losing weight. Her clothes were too big and the scale showed lower and lower readings. Brenda was getting results and she knew it. However, anytime someone complimented Brenda on her weight loss, she would frown and say things like: "You think so? I don't see it." Or, "Yeah, but, I'm still fat." Or, "I still have such a long way to go." Brenda talked about herself the way cast members who don't like each other talk on a negative reality TV show. Despite her clearly noticeable improvements, Brenda criticized herself in a disparaging way that was disrespectful to herself and her progress. After a while, Brenda started to eat the pizza again, drink soda and she stopped exercising.

Brenda did not RESPECT the results she was getting. Brenda's downfall can and will be your downfall if you do what Brenda did. Brenda's lack of respect for her fitness accomplishments discouraged her enough to make her stop doing the things that were helping her. Brenda lacked respect for the discipline it took for her not to eat so much pizza or drink as much soda. Brenda's lack of respect for her restraint and body transformation discouraged her enough to make her stop doing the things that were helping her. If you do not add respect into your fitness program, then it is likely that you will not maintain your fitness results either.

Your fitness journey may start with a deal you make with yourself, such as, you'll stop eating or drinking this or that in exchange for a smaller waist line, more toned arms, or a firmer booty. Respect your process to become fit. Respect the results you get throughout your process. And, realize the deal you make with yourself to be more fit will be broken when there is a lack of respect for the process of transforming your body and a lack of respect for any positive results you obtain throughout the process.

The best news in all of this is that it is easy to start *respecting* you, your process and your results (small or great).

You are special and your body is very valuable. As with many things that are valuable, you may need to consult with experts to get special instructions on how to deal with your body. Thus, be a wise fit mama and educate yourself about fitness, food and your body's specific response to fitness and food. Be positive about learning from health and fitness experts who are trained in this area.

You may have to make a financial contribution to your fitness education and better health pursuits. But, understand that you are worth every penny. The alternative cost of medication and unhealthy fast food making you feel less than your best is just not worth it. Your children will certainly appreciate having a mama who invest in herself, is more active and has more energy and stamina for them.

Lastly, obstacles are going to come. Setbacks to your fitness goals may happen. A victory today can mean a defeat tomorrow, so always press ahead to your health & fitness goals and pay for help if necessary. If you respect the process and the results you get (small or great) along the way, then you are well on the path to being a fit mama with a rocking body!

# THE THREE P'STHAT WILL HELP YOU TO SUCCEED

### BY KARLA WALKER

**These 3 Components Will Get You A Rocking Body That Will Make Everyone Say-WOW!**

What Brenda did to act on the information in chapter nine best illustrates the three essential points for this chapter: 1. Staying Positive. 2. Keep Pressing. 3. Remain patient. A couple of months after Brenda got discouraged about her fitness program, she gained all of her weight back and more. Brenda stopped the candle light dinners for her husband and wearing the lingerie that gave her U.S. Marine husband a hero's welcome after his tour of duty. At times, Brenda stopped feeling shamed by all of the weight she gained and she managed to be intimate with her husband. But, Brenda had strict love making stipulations, which included but are not limited to: no undressing in front of her husband, keeping all the lights off, and never being positioned on top (so her husband would not have to see what she called her saddlebag breast and an ocean wave of fat rolls). At all cost, Brenda hid her body.

After while, Brenda's children had to stop their extra curricular activities because she no longer had the energy to deal with the hustle and bustle of their schedule. Brenda was too tired.

One day, Brenda received an unsettling report from the pediatrician that her, now rotund, young sons were overweight for their age. And, they were at an increased risk of having Type II Diabetes within the year if they did not make immediate dietary changes. But, the most heartbreaking part for Brenda was having to wipe the tears from her daughter's newly pudgy face as she retold Brenda the daily teasing and bullying she endured at her elementary school for being overweight. Brenda sat down with her children to see if they would be interested in getting back involved in their former active lifestyle. Brenda was saddened and feeling guilty as she listened to her children call themselves fat and other negative things. But, Brenda was hesitant to correct them because she had said the same things about herself.

One thing was very clear to Brenda as she sat listening to her children say the same degrading jokes about themselves. Brenda was having a defining moment.

Was Brenda going to keep being a spectator to her and her children's weight gain? Was Brenda going to reverse her and her children's poor health into good health? Was Brenda going to have her and her children discouraged and defeated by the lie that they will never be fit? Well, the warrior inside of Brenda that gave her the strength to give birth to these three beautiful children rose up and shouted-ENOUGH! Her children looked at Brenda in anticipation of what she was going to say. Brenda began to speak candidly from her heart to her children of how unhappy she is with the condition of her body and how she wants to get healthy and fit. She asked them to join her with being in better health. To Brenda's surprise, her children agreed.

Brenda researched for a Personal Trainer who was knowledgeable, experienced and who could hold her accountable in a way that was professional and motivating to Brenda. Brenda's co-worker had a personal trainer for years. She told Brenda to make sure she found a personal trainer that she liked as a outside of person. Brenda's co-worker's personal trainer was not going to work for Brenda. Fortunately, Brenda found a personal trainer that could train her online and and in person when time permitted.

Her personal trainer helped Brenda act on the three P's of a Fit Mama.

**Number One: Positivity**

Always see the glass as half full concerning being a healthy and fit mama. You should strive to be your most consistent cheerleader on your journey to a rocking body. Protect yourselves from negativity by teaching your children and love ones to be positive about your health and fitness goals. For example, tell your kids and friends not to tempt you with junk food. And, lastly on this point, treat discouragement as an acquaintance not a best friend. You will encounter discouragement, but just as you do not hangout regularly with an acquaintance, do not hangout with or entertain discouragement for long periods of time as though discouragement is your best friend. *Positivity is an important part of your journey!*

## Number Two: Pressing

Another way to say stay driven toward meeting your goal of being a fit mama is to say keep pressing. One way to keep pressing on your journey of becoming a fit mama is by getting involved in healthy competition. This may mean participating in a local 5K walk/run or a health challenge at your office. These activities can keep you motivated to press toward your goals and finish strong.

Fit mama, make a decision to press through your workouts. Press through for the love of yourself, your children and your spouse/companion. Good workouts will give you the energy and stamina you need to enjoy your life individually as a woman and collectively as a mom and partner. Lastly, some moms just focus on losing weight, as though being a thin mom is the best mom. But, did you know that skinny people are in the hospital beds and die too. I say that to say: do not just focus on looking healthy, but press to actually be healthy-inside and out. This may mean investing in supplements, alternative health treatments, exercise, etc., that will address your internal and external health. *Pressing toward your goal of a Fit Mama inside and out is essential to your journey!*

## And, Number Three: Patient

Be patient with yourself and your body as you get healthy and fit. You may have to be like Brenda and others who choose to invest in themselves by hiring a Personal Trainer or purchase natural health and fitness services. Be patient with the supplements and/or equipment you may purchase to help you get results. And, be patient with the process of transforming your health and physique. Always remember, wherever you start on your health journey took time to get this way and it will take time to get lasting results. And, candidly speaking, even if you were to get the body you want overnight, you will need longer than one night to learn your new body and what you need to do in order to maintain your results. So, all in all, be patient. You need patience on your journey for better health for yourselves, kids, spouse/partner and loved ones.

~So, Remember Your Time to have a Rocking Optimal Body is Now! ~

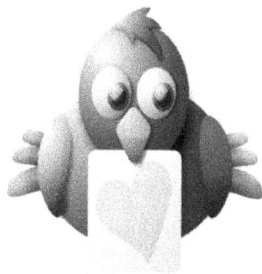

**Karla and Rich's Personal Training Tips #7:** Fit Mamas are positive, pressing toward their goals and patient with themselves.

**Final Book Bonus: Mom-Minded Fitness Plan #7:** Have a romantic walk in the park with yourself. One of my most favorite memories of Rich and I was when we were dating and we took a long walk through this really nice park. We talked, enjoyed the beauty of nature and focused on many positive aspects of our relationship. Fortunately, Rich and I still make time for moments like this, just not at the same park. And, I expanded this quite therapeutic activity into a reward I give myself for my hard workouts and compliance to my nutritional plan. For example, I may find time during a run to stop, walk, and enjoy the beauty of nature and the many positive aspects of my health and fitness program. I return home feeling renewed, encouraged and empowered to be a happier Fit Mama. This activity also reiterates a healthy message we teach our children, which is learn to be happy with yourself and let others add to the happiness you already have inside. So…

Mom-minded Fitness Plan #7 is for you to make time for your own stroll where you can just love yourself and appreciate your fitness progress and life.

**Final Thoughts**

*Karla and Rich's Personal Training Tip #:*

1. Fit Mamas speak motivating words about their fitness efforts.

2. Fit Mamas learn their body-type and body-shape and are encouraged.

3. Fit Mamas set goals for their body-type and body-shape.

4. Fit Mamas gladly examine their fitness routine and make adjustments to stay on their fitness program.

5. Fit Mamas make it a priority to put themselves on their agenda.

6. Fit Mamas always challenging themselves.

7. Fit Mamas are positive, pressing toward their goals and patient with themselves.

You make sacrifices everyday as a loving mom. As a mom, you motivate your children to walk, talk, to be creative and more. We learn ways to help them; whether, it is potty training, little league/ school, you help your children set and reach their goals. From babies and beyond, as a mom you examine their development and make adjustments, so they will improve. Your children are a priority that stays on your agenda. You challenge them to be the best and enjoy life. Lastly, as it concerns your children, your love for them keeps you positive, pressing them toward their goals and dreams, and keeps you patient to never give up on your kids. So, as a mom, you have what is needed to get and stay fit. Allow the love you have toward your children to ricochet to you, so you can apply these seven secrets of a fit mama to your life in order for you to be a fit mama too!

In good health~

Karla and Rich Walker

*Find us on Facebook, Twitter, and YouTube. We would enjoy connecting with you. If you want your thoughts about this book posted on our website to encourage other mamas like you, submit your comment and photo (if desired) on our website:* **www.richandkarlawalker.com**

# ABOUT THE AUTHORS

Rich and Karla Walker are Health and Fitness Experts with a *combined* 71 years of professional experience in the areas of physical health, mental health, and spiritual health. Thus, their personal and professional qualifications assist them in providing expert advice and guidance on matters relating to health and wellness of the total person (spiritually, mentally, emotionally, and physically).

Mr. and Mrs. Walker have been best friends for over 16 years. They spend significant amounts of quality time together, and they still enjoy each other's company just as much as they did on their wedding day and honeymoon. They are grateful for their partnership and are happily and successfully married with six children conceived together. Their sixth child was born on August 27, 2014.

Lastly, the Walkers have appeared on Fox 2 News- Detroit's Fox Affiliate, 7 Action News - Detroit's ABC Affiliate, The Detroit News, The Detroit Free Press, The Oakland Press, The Michigan Chronicle, The Michigan Front Page, Crain's Detroit Business, 950 AM on The Murray Feldman Report, Wake Up Detroit with Former Detroit City Councilwoman Joann Watson, 1200 AM WCHB, and more.